Complications of Bone Marrow and Stem Cell Transplants: Fast Focus Study Guide

JT Thomas, MD

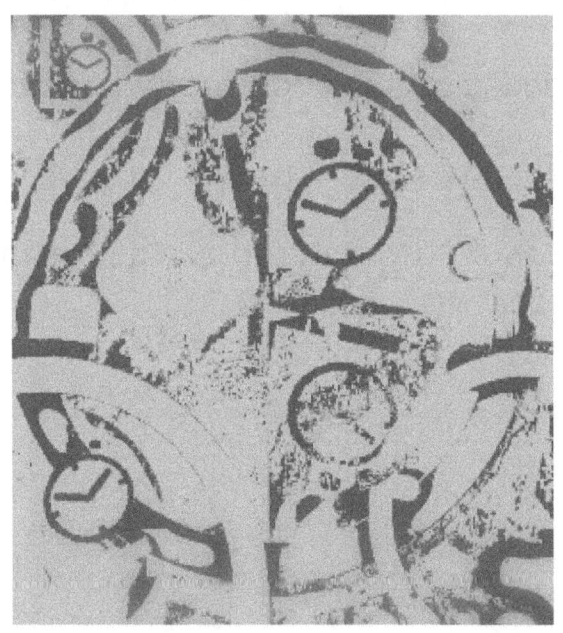

Acknowledgements

I dedicate this book to my beautiful wife and children, who I love more than all the water in all the oceans and all the seas.

CONTENTS

- This book is written to help the reader further understand the process and complications of bone marrow and stem cell transplants.

- This book is written in a simple and easy to read format.

- This book simplifies a complicated medical issue so you will remember the important details.

- You will not get caught up in the minutia.

- This Fast Focus Study Guide will provide you with a practical review of the key information you need to know.

- Buy this book now if you want this quick and concise information

The Basics of HLA Matching

and Transplantation

It is important to understand HLA antigens and their role in bone marrow transplant. HLA antigens are inherited as a group. Each of us have two groups of HLA antigens (one we received from our father and the other we received from our mother). Each sibling has a 25% chance of having the same HLA haplotype (HLA-A, -B, -C, -DR, -DQ, and -DP). Each parent will have one HLA haplotype in common with each of their children.

When matching bone marrow, at least 8 HLA markers are evaluated: two A markers, two B markers, two C markers, and two DRB1 markers. Sometimes the DQ proteins are matched. An adult donor needs to match at least 6 of the 8 HLA markers to be compatible for transplantation. Since cord blood has a less mature immune system, most centers require that at least 4 of 6 markers match at HLA-A, -B, and -DRB1.

Class I antigens are composed of two chains and include HLA-A, -B, and -C antigens. Class I antigens are basically found on every cell in the body.

Class II antigens are composed of two polymorphic chains and include DR, DQ, and DP antigens. Class II antigens are found on B-cells. These antigens are sometimes induced to be expressed on other cells in the setting of injury or inflammation.

About 70% of patients who need a transplant do not have a HLA matched donor in their family. In that situation an unrelated donor or cord blood unit is found.

About 30% of patients are able to find an unrelated donor. Cord blood can be obtained quicker than a matched unrelated donor donation. The immune system of the patient (infant) who donated the cord blood has an undeveloped immune system and therefore graft-versus-host disease (GVHD) is less common than what is seen even with related or unrelated donors.

Cord blood transplantation is associated with a slow rate of engraftment and prolonged myelosuppression and neutropenia with delayed immune reconstitution,   This is associated with higher mortality from infection. Up to 10% of patients fail to engraft. Haploidentical and cord blood transplants have similar success rates.

Patients sometimes cannot find a fully matched HLA donor. If there are no other options, a haploidentical donor can be used. That means that one of the two groups of HLA antigens are a match. Parents are always haploidentical with their children, and siblings have a 50% chance of being haploidentical with each other. About 90% of patients will have a haploidentical donor.

Haploidentical transplantation is characterized by a high rate of severe acute GVHD and delayed immune reconstitution. The rate of acute GVHD can be decreased by T-cell depletion, immunosuppression, and post-transplantation chemotherapy with cyclophosphamide or bortezomib.

Peripheral blood stem cell transplants are much more common than the traditional bone marrow transplant. In a stem cell transplant cytokines and chemotherapy stimulate stem cells out of the bone marrow and into the peripheral blood. Leukapharesis is started when the CD34 cell count exceeds 5-10 cells/mL.

Peripheral blood collection of stem cells is more common now because stem cell collection is much easier and less invasive. Additionally, the recipient blood count recovers is faster with the stem cells than the bone marrow transplant.

Plerixafor aids in stem cell recovery from the peripheral blood. It is an antagonist of CXCR4 that causes a rapid and increase in the total WBC and peripheral blood CD34 counts at 4 and 6 hours after a single injection. Currently G-CSF is used in combination with plerixafor. Plerixafor is associated with gastrointestinal disorders and injection site reactions.

Allogeneic peripheral blood stem cell transplant is characterized by a faster neutrophil recovery and higher rates of chronic GVHD.

Some patients cannot tolerate or do not need high dose chemotherapy prior to transplant. The scientists have developed reduced-intensity conditioning regimens that are associated with decreased nonhematologic toxicities and a transient mixed chimerism after transplant.

Total body irradiation administered prior to bone marrow/stem cell transplant is associated with pulmonary toxicity, cataract formation, and thyroid dysfunction.

BuCy administered prior to bone marrow/stem cell transplant is associated with a higher incidence of veno-occlusive disease (VOD) and irreversible alopecia.

Reduced-intensity conditioning regimens have are characterized by the dose of the chemotherapy: melphalan <150 mg/m2;busulfan < 9mg/kg of the oral equivalent; thiotepa <10 mg/kg; and TBI <500 cGy single fraction or 800 cGy fractionated.

Graft Versus Host Disease

Graft versus host disease develops when the donor bone marrow immune system identifies the donor recipient as foreign. The activated donor immune system most often affects the skin, GI tract and liver.

Acute GVHD is present < 100 days after the transplant. Chronic GVHD is present > 100 days after transplant.

The risk for GVHD increases if the patient undergoing the transplant had a donor that was from an HLA mismatched related donor (or from an HLA matched unrelated donor). The risk for GVHD also increases if there is a female donor who has been pregnant in the past. Additional risk factors include an advanced age of either the donor or the recipient, or if there is inadequate immunosuppression.

Symptoms of acute GVHD include fever, elevated liver tests, rash, nausea, diarrhea, abdominal pain, and weight loss.

Chronic GVHD is said to occur if the patient is more than 100 days out from transplant. It may manifest as a continuation of acute GVHD or occur after acute GVHD has resolved.

Chronic GVHD often affects primarily the skin and can show up as a lichenoid rash or with scleroderma type symptoms. If it affects mucous membranes it can be characterized as keratoconjunctivitis sicca, periodontitis, orogenital lichenoid reactions. This disorder can affect the GI tract, liver, and lungs where it can manifest as bronchiolitis obliterans.

Prophylaxis for GVHD commonly combines a calcineurin inhibitor (cyclosporine or tacrolimus) with methotrexate. Sirolimus and mycophenolate mofetil are often used instead of methotrexate secondary to the mucosal and kidney toxicities associated with methotrexate.

GVHD prevention can be accomplished with graft T-cell depletion with T-cell depleting treatments such as ATG and alemtuzumab. This approach is associated with increased rate of infections secondary to the additional immunosuppression.

Treatment of acute GVHD corticosteroids, at 2 mg/kg/d with calcineurin inhibitors (tacrolimus, cyclosporine).

Treatment for chronic GVHD (>100 days from transplant) consists of corticosteroids alone. Studies have shown that combinations of corticosteroids with other medications such as azathioprine or cyclosporine are not better than steroids alone.

Immunosuppression can be stopped 6 months after HSC transplantation if no chronic GVHD has developed.

Bone Marrow/Stem Cell Transplantation and CMV

CMV infections are most important viral cause of illness and death after allogeneic bone marrow transplant.

CMV infection in bone marrow transplant patients are characterized by fever, fatigue, thrombocytopenia, leukopenia, elevated liver tests.

Ganciclovir alone is the first line treatment for CMV gastroenteritis, retinitis or other disease manifestation. The treatment for CMV pneumonia is ganiciclovir in combination with IVIG.

Bone marrow transplant recipient seropositivity indicates the presence of latent CMV infection and is the most important risk factor for CMV disease after transplant.

Bone marrow transplant recipient seropositivity indicates the presence of latent CMV infection and is the most important risk factor for CMV disease after transplant.

Patients who are CMV negative recipients of a bone marrow transplant from a CMV positive donor are less likely to have CMV disease than a patient who is CMV positive who receives a bone marrow transplant from a CMV negative patient.

CMV disease is most likely to occur 1-3 months after bone marrow transplant.

CMV infections occur in 60-70% of bone marrow recipients who are CMV positive prior to transplant regardless of whether the donor is CMV positive or negative.

CMV infections occur in about 30% of bone

marrow recipients who are CMV negative

who have a CMV positive donor.

CMV infection occurs most commonly around

day 40 after bone marrow transplantation.

CMV pneumonitis most commonly occurs
around day 55 after bone marrow
transplantation.

CMV pneumonia has an untreated mortality in the range of 80% and presents with fever, nonproductive cough, hypoxia, and interstitial infiltrates on chest radiograph.

CMV pneumonitis should be treated with ganiciclovir plus immunoglobulin since treatment with ganciclovir or foscarnet alone is considered inferior.

CMV negative or leuko-reduced blood should be used for CMV negative allogeneic BMT recipients, even if the donor was CMV positive.

Prophylactic ganciclovir reduces CMV infection but does not improve survival following allogeneic BMT in CMV positive patients.

CMV positive patients receiving bone marrow transplants from unrelated or HLA-mismatched donors are at very high risk of developing CMV disease.

Low risk patients for CMV disease who have a CMV positive donor or who are a CMV positive recipient should be monitored weekly for at least 100 days (sometimes longer) after the transplant with either the CMV antigen assay or PCR.

Testing for CMV antibodies (IgG and IgM) is not effective in diagnosing post transplant infection and is used only to determine patients risk for developing infection post transplant.

Herpes Simplex Virus Infection

Herpes simplex virus reactivation will occur in absence of viral prophylaxis in 60-70% of HSV positive bone marrow transplant recipients in the setting of chemotherapy-induced neutropenia and mucositis.

If HSV prophylaxis is not given after bone marrow transplant HSV reactivation can occur in up to 80% of seropositive disease.

HSV prophylaxis with acyclovir or valacyclovir is started with bone marrow conditioning therapy and continued until engraftment.

HSV infection is characterized by mucositis, genital herpes, esophagitis or pneumonia.

HSV typically presents within 2 - 3 weeks of bone marrow transplant and is mainly due to reactivation for the latent virus.

Risk of HSV reactivation potential need for prophylaxis with bone marrow transplant is dependent on serologic status of the bone marrow transplant recipient.

Acyclovir prophylaxis is not indicated for HSV-seronegative bone marrow transplant recipients, even if the donor is HSV seropositive.

Foscarnet is the drug of choice for resistant HSV infection.

Herpes simplex virus infections characterized by severe localized infections or those characterized as having visceral or disseminated after allogeneic transplant should be treated with IV acyclovir.

Herpes simplex virus infections characterized as less severe mucocutaneous disease can be treated with oral acyclovir.

Herpes Simplex positive bone marrow transplant recipients who are not receiving prophylactic ganciclovir should receive acyclovir prophylaxis (iv or oral) from the beginning of conditioning for a period of 4 weeks . Of note, ganciclovir prophylaxis against CMV disease also protects against herpes simplex reactivation.

Varicella Zoster virus infections that develop within 12 months of bone marrow transplant. If the patient has had a transplant and is on immunosuppressive treatment, they should receive IV acyclovir is the treatment of choice.

Human Herpes Virus

Infection

Human Herpes virus 6 is associated with pneumonitis, encephalitis and self-limiting symptoms following bone marrow transplant.

Most cases of human herpes virus 6 infection after bone marrow transplant occurs as a consequence of viral reactivation.

human herpes virus 6 reactivation occurs in
40 - 60 % of patients after bone marrow
transplant who were seropositive prior to
bone marrow transplant.

It is important to know that human herpes virus 6 reactivation after bone marrow transplant often manifests as HHV-6 encephalitis.

There is some data that HHV 7 infection in the post-transplant patient is associated with delayed neutrophil engraftment.

HHV-8 causes Kaposi's sarcoma which is not common in the setting of bone marrow transplant.

Engraftment Syndrome

Engraftment Syndrome is characterized by dyspnea, fever and erythematous maculo-papular rash and organ dysfunction.

Engraftment Syndrome is associated with increased capillary leak and typically presents 7-12 days post after bone marrow transplant and within 4 days of granulocyte recovery.

It is important to know that engraftment syndrome is seen more commonly in autologous bone marrow transplant than in allogeneic bone marrow transplant.

Engraftment syndrome is treated with corticosteroids.

Diffuse Alveolar Hemorrhage

Diffuse Alveolar Hemorrhage (DAH) is characterized by onset of dyspnea, cough, fever, and hypoxemia occurring at a median of 21-23.5 days after either an allogenic or autologous bone marrow transplant.

Diffuse Alveolar Hemorrhage (DAH) is associated with infection and diffuse alveolar damage and is characterized by chest imaging showing patchy or diffuse opacities with air bronchograms progressing to a diffuse alveolar pattern.

Diffuse Alveolar Hemorrhage (DAH) is diagnosed with lung biopsy demonstrating pure blood in at least 30% of the evaluated alveolar surface area.

Diffuse alveolar hemorrhage has a mortality of 70–100%. Patients with onset prior to 30 days after transplant have a better prognosis than those with onset more than 30 days after transplant.

Risk factors for diffuse alveolar hemorrhage include age greater than 40 years, intensity of preparative regime, infection, thrombocytopenia, and GVHD.

Diffuse alveolar hemorrhage is treated with high-dose corticosteroids. Mortality is decreased when aminocaproic acid is added to high dose methylprednisolone.

Hepatic Sinusoidal

Obstruction

(Veno-Occlusive Disease)

Hepatic sinusoidal obstruction syndrome (hepatic veno-occlusive disease) is characterized by hepatomegaly and abdominal pain. Patients also develop jaundice, fluid retention with weight gain > 10% and ascites.

Hepatic sinusoidal obstruction syndrome is caused by the preparative regimen toxicity endothelial injury in both sinusoids and small hepatic venules with intrahepatic thrombosis with centrilobular hemorrhagic necrosis. Patients develop liver failure and coagulopathy.

There is increased risk of developing hepatic sinusoidal obstruction syndrome (VOD) in patients with a history of underlying hepatocellular damage which can develop after treatements such as TBI and exposures to toxic drugs (busulfan, carmustine, gemtuzumab).

Hepatic sinusoidal obstruction syndrome (VOD) can be treated with an adenosine receptor agonist called defibrotide.

Hepatic sinusoidal obstruction syndrome low-dose heparin and ursodiol.

━━━━━━━━━━━━━━━━━━━━━━━━━━━━━

Mucositis

Mucositis affects about 75% of the patients who undergo chemotherapy or total body irradiation prior to bone marrow transplant.

Mucositis develops 7 to 10 days after initiation of high-dose chemotherapy or total body irradiation prior to bone marrow transplant.

Palifermin is a keratinocyte growth factor that decreases the development and severity of severe oral mucositis in patients with hematologic cancers receiving high-dose chemotherapy and/or radiation therapy for bone marrow transplantation.

Patients are given three daily doses of palifermin before chemotherapy/radiation and three additional daily doses starting on the day of transplant.

Mucositis can be complicated by infection and generally heals within 2 to 4 weeks.

Post-Transplant

Lymphoproliferative Disorder

EBV Post-transplant lymphoproliferative disease (EBV-PTLD) is a heterogeneous disease that can be quite aggressive with a predilection for CNS and visceral involvement.

PTLD is a typically a high grade lymphoma characterized by EBV-transformed B cells that develop in the absence of controlling T cells due to T cell depletion and immunosuppressants.

PTLD most commonly develops within the first post-transplant year.

EBV-negative PTLD can occur but generally develops later than those that are EBV positive with a median time from transplant to PTLD of 50-60 months vs. 6 months in EBV positive. EBV negative PTLD is associated with a poor prognosis.

Post-transplant lymphoproliferative disorders (PTLD) can occur in patients who have received solid organ, bone marrow, or stem cell transplant.

The risk of developing PTLD is proportional to the degree of required immunosuppression and therefore depends on the conditioning regimen and the required T-cell depletion.

PTLD is associated with Epstein-Barr virus (EBV) infection of B cells secondary to viral reactivation or primary EBV infection.

EBV DNA load may rise as early as three weeks before PTLD onset. Patients can be considered high risk by monitoring EBV DNA load with quantitative PCR.

The majority of PTLDs in solid organ recipients are of transplant recipient origin and the majority of PTLDs in bone marrow transplant recipients are of donor origin.

Some patients will respond to a reduction in immunosuppressive drugs but most will need additional systemic therapy.

The median time for PTLD to respond to treatment is approximately 1 month.

Single-agent rituximab is well tolerated and has an overall response rate of 40% to 75% with a the 1-year overall survival in the range of 60-70%.

The PTLD-adapted prognostic score can be helpful in determining which patients are high risk. High risk patients likely will need treatment in addition to single agent Rituxan. This score incorporates age (>60 years), elevated LDH, and PS (>2). Patients who had a score of 0 had an overall 2 year survival of 88%. A score of 1 had a 2 year survival of 50%, and a score of 2 or 3 had a 2 year survival of 0%.

If reduced immunosuppression and single-agent rituximab does not yield a complete remission then sequential therapy with R-CHOP can be used up front with G-CSF support with strong consideration also for PCP prophylaxis for patients who present with very high risk disease.

There is some data using donor-derived, EBV-specific cytotoxic T- Lymphocytes to prevent PTLD in patients who have received T-cell-depleted unrelated or mismatched allogeneic transplants.

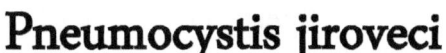

Pneumocystis jiroveci

Pneumocystis jiroveci causes fungal pneumonia in immunocompromised patients with a median onset at 9 weeks after transplant.

The risk of Pneumocystis jiroveci pneumonia is greatest in the first 6 months after transplantation however late onset PCP also is known to occur in patients after discontinuing prophylaxis more than 6 months out from transplant.

The risk of Pneumocystis jiroveci pneumonia is increased in patients receiving T cell depleted bone marrow or those diagnosed with chronic GVHD.

Pneumocystis jiroveci pneumonia prophylaxis is accomplished with oral trimethoprim/sulfamethoxazole or inhaled pentamidine.

Trimethoprin/sulfamethoxazole also provides prophylaxis against toxoplasma, Streptococcus pneumonia and other community-acquired pneumonia.

Pneumocystis jirovecii Pneumonia prophylaxis is typically administered until completion of immune suppression and recovery of the immune system characterized by a CD4 >200.

Candida albicans is the most common fungal pathogen during the pre-engraftment period however, after engraftment, the most common fungal infection is invasive Aspergillosis.

The risk of developing fungal infection after bone marrow transplant is directly related to the duration of neutropenia. This begins to increase after approximately 5-7 days of neutropenia.

The risk for invasive Aspergillosis after bone marrow transplant is increased in the setting of GVHD and prolonged corticosteroids.

Bone marrow transplant recipients account for 32% of all Aspergillus infections.

Drug Toxicity

Cyclosporine is a calcineurin inhibitor used for immunosuppression in patients undergoing bone marrow/stem cell transplant. The most common side effects include nephrotoxicity, hypertension, hyperkalemia, hypomagnesemia, hyperuricemia, headache, tremors, leg cramps, convulsions, hirsutism, acne, nausea/vomiting, abdominal pain, diarrhea, and gingival hyperplasia.

Tacrolimus is a macrolide calcineurin inhibitor used for immunosuppression in patients undergoing bone marrow/stem cell transplant. The most common side effects include hypertension, fluid retention, diarrhea, hyperglycemia, anemia, headache, tremor, insomnia, pain, and asthenia, nephrotoxicity, hyperkalemia (or hypokalemia), and hypomagnesemia.

Mycophenolate mofetil reversibly inhibits inosine monophosphate dehydrogenase and prevents lymphocyte proliferation that is used for immunosuppression in patients undergoing bone marrow/stem cell transplant. The most common side effects include upset stomach, nausea, vomiting or diarrhea. Patients are at increased risk of opportunistic infections including shingles, herpes, cytomegalovirus, and BK virus associated nephropathy. Mycophenolate is also associated progressive multifocal leukoencephalopathy.

Sirolimus prevents activation of T and B cells by inhibiting IL-2. that is used for immunosuppression in patients undergoing bone marrow/stem cell transplant. Patients using this medication are at increased risk for infections and lymphoma, impaired wound healing, hypercholesterolemia and hypertriglyceridemia, hypertension, thrombocytopenia and to a lesser extent anemia, arthralgia, acne and rash, increased risk of interstitial pneumonitis, upper respiratory tract infections, insomnia and tremor.

Foscarnet is a DNA phosphorylation inhibitor used to treat resistant HSV and ganciclovir-resistant viruses. Foscarnet has to be renally dosed and is nephrotoxic. This medication can alter calcium and phosphorus metabolism. Other potential side effects include anemia, headache, nausea, neurologic side effects and a fixed drug reaction involving the penis.

Ganciclovir is a nucleoside analogue that inhibits DNA synthesis in the same manner as acyclovir. Acyclovir does not work for CMV because CMV does not contain a thymidine kinase. Ganciclovir has activity against CMV, HSV, VZV, and HHV-6, HHV-7, and HHV-8. The major adverse effects of ganciclovir therapy include fever, rash, diarrhea, neutropenia, anemia, thrombocytopenia.

Voriconazole is a broad-spectrum triazole that is the treatment of choice for Aspergillus infections. Adverse effects that must be monitored for include hepatotoxicity, visual disturbances, hallucinations, dermatologic reactions, and QT prolongation.

Posaconazole is a triazole that effectively treats yeast and mold including various dematiaceous fungi. It is the only oral azole effective against many of the species that cause mucormycosis. It can be used for fungal prophylaxis in neutropenic patients. Side effects include a QT prolongation, hepatitis, nausea, mild diarrhea, abdominal discomfort, indigestion and dry mouth, skin rash, fever, fatigue, and loss of appetite.

Itraconazole is a synthetic triazole used to treat lymphocutaneous sporotrichosis, histoplasmosis, blastomycosis, and paracoccidioidomycosis. It is also effective in mild cases of invasive aspergillosis, some cases of coccidioidomycosis, and chromoblastomycosis. Common side effects are nausea and sickness, occasional abdominal discomfort, constipation, fluid retention, rashes, and abnormal liver function tests. The FDA has issued a black box warning for heart failure.

Fluconazole is a bis-triazole used to treat Candida species (not Candida krusei or Candida glabrata). It is active against other yeasts and no activity against Aspergillus. It is absorbed almost completely after an oral dose. It is excreted essentially unchanged in urine.

It has high penetration into CSF ($\geq$ 70% of serum levels) and has been especially useful in treating cryptococcal and coccidioidal meningitis. Common side effects include GI discomfort and rash. Other potential toxicity include hepatic necrosis, Stevens-Johnson syndrome, anaphylaxis.

This concludes Complications of Bone Marrow and Stem Cell Transplants:
Fast Focus Study Guide

Search Amazon or other book retailers to find other books in the
Fast Focus Study Guide Series

Search Amazon Print Books and Kindle books to find other study guides written by
JT Thomas, MD

Internal Medicine Study Guide

Hematology Study Guide

Medical Oncology Study Guide

Cardiology Study Guide

Nephrology Study Guide

Multiple Myeloma Study Guide

Differential Diagnosis Study Guide

Ovarian Cancer Study Guide

Rheumatology Study Guide

Cancer Study Guide